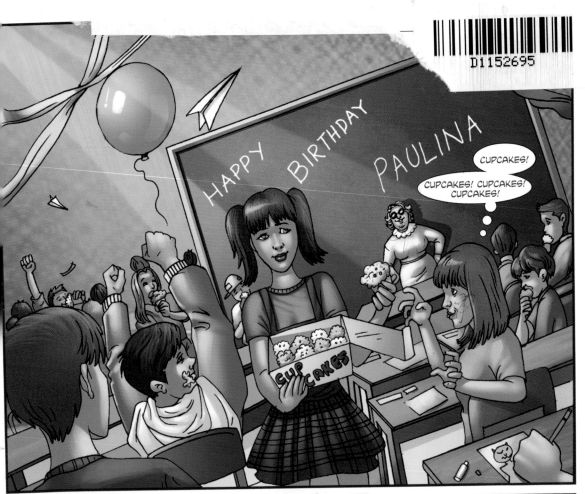

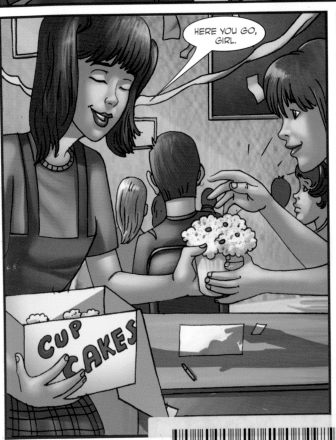

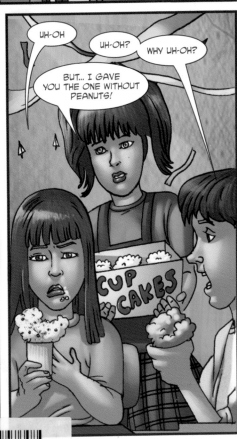

1

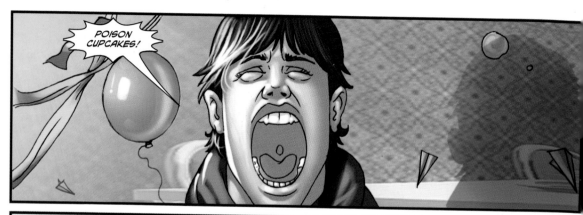

POISON CUPCAKES!

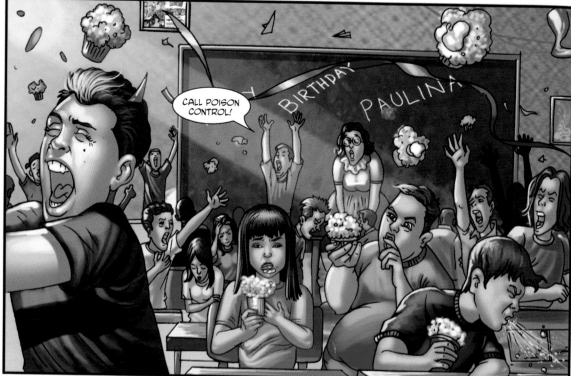

CALL POISON CONTROL!

BIRTHDAY PAULINA

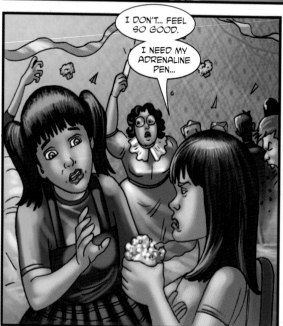

I DON'T... FEEL SO GOOD.

I NEED MY ADRENALINE PEN...

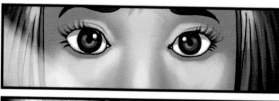

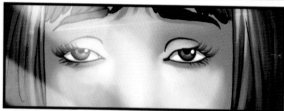

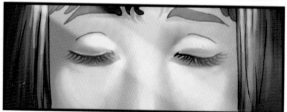

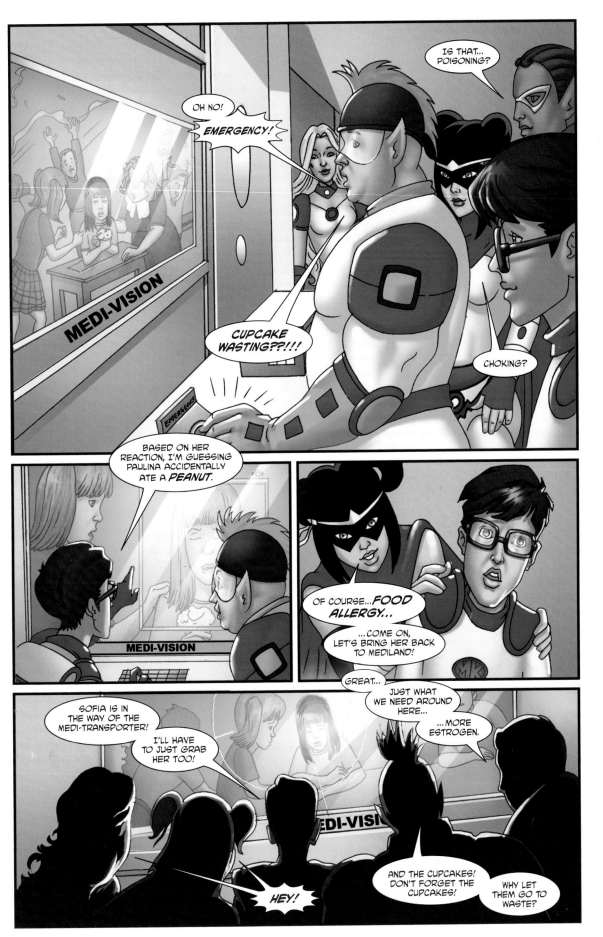

3

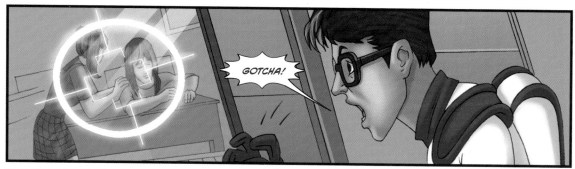

GOTCHA!

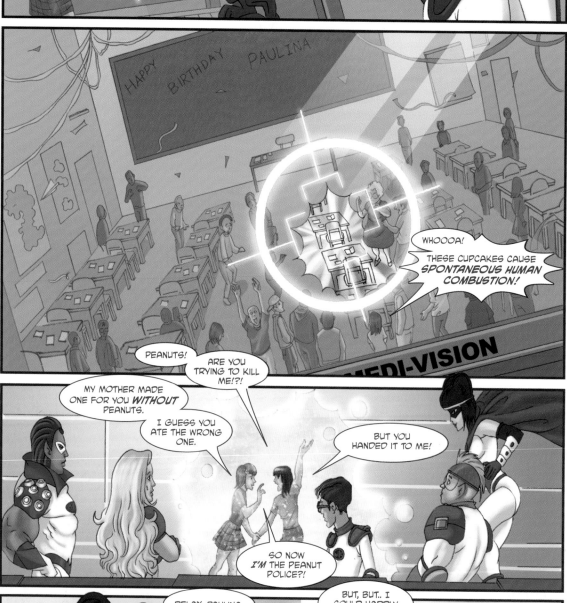

HAPPY BIRTHDAY PAULINA

WHOOOA! THESE CUPCAKES CAUSE *SPONTANEOUS HUMAN COMBUSTION!*

MEDI-VISION

PEANUTS! ARE YOU TRYING TO KILL ME!?!

MY MOTHER MADE ONE FOR YOU *WITHOUT* PEANUTS.

I GUESS YOU ATE THE WRONG ONE.

BUT YOU HANDED IT TO ME!

SO NOW *I'M* THE PEANUT POLICE?!

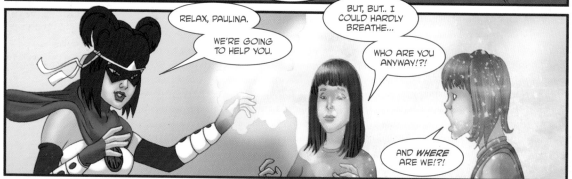

RELAX, PAULINA.

WE'RE GOING TO HELP YOU.

BUT, BUT.. I COULD HARDLY BREATHE...

WHO ARE YOU ANYWAY!?!

AND *WHERE* ARE WE!?!

4

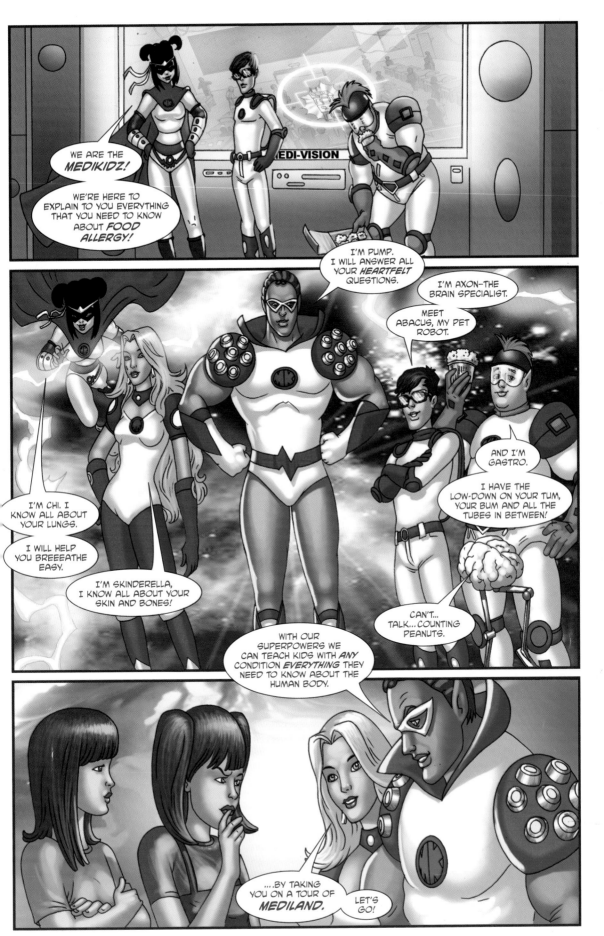

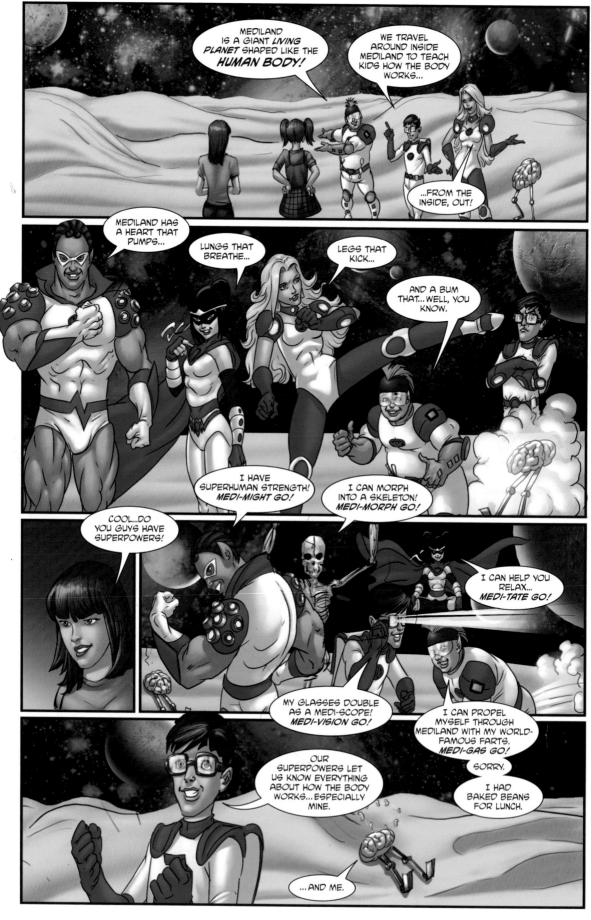

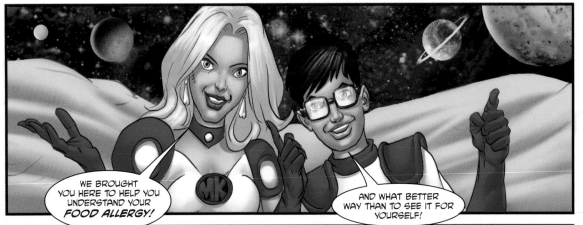

WE BROUGHT YOU HERE TO HELP YOU UNDERSTAND YOUR *FOOD ALLERGY!*

AND WHAT BETTER WAY THAN TO SEE IT FOR YOURSELF!

FOOD ALLERGY... I GET IT!

DON'T EAT ANYTHING THAT TASTES GOOD!

YOU MAY AS WELL JUST SEND US HOME NOW.

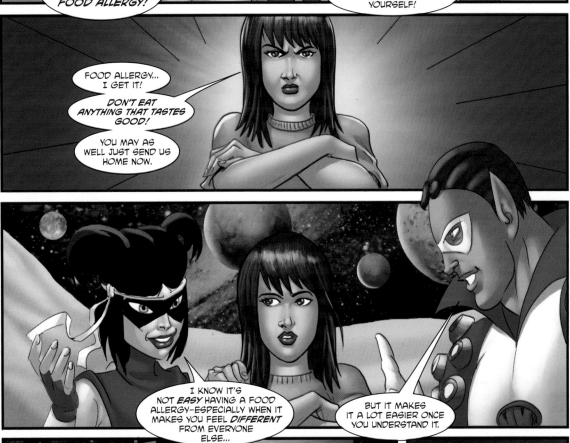

I KNOW IT'S NOT *EASY* HAVING A FOOD ALLERGY—ESPECIALLY WHEN IT MAKES YOU FEEL *DIFFERENT* FROM EVERYONE ELSE...

BUT IT MAKES IT A LOT EASIER ONCE YOU UNDERSTAND IT.

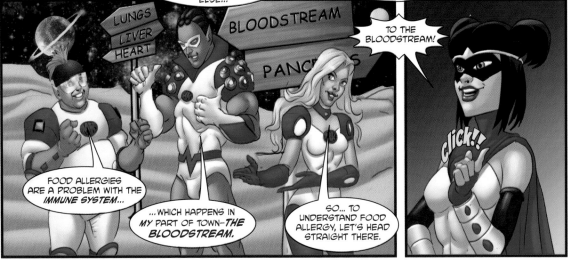

LUNGS
LIVER
HEART

BLOODSTREAM

PANCREAS

TO THE BLOODSTREAM!

FOOD ALLERGIES ARE A PROBLEM WITH THE *IMMUNE SYSTEM*...

...WHICH HAPPENS IN *MY PART OF TOWN—THE BLOODSTREAM.*

SO... TO UNDERSTAND FOOD ALLERGY, LET'S HEAD STRAIGHT THERE.

click!!

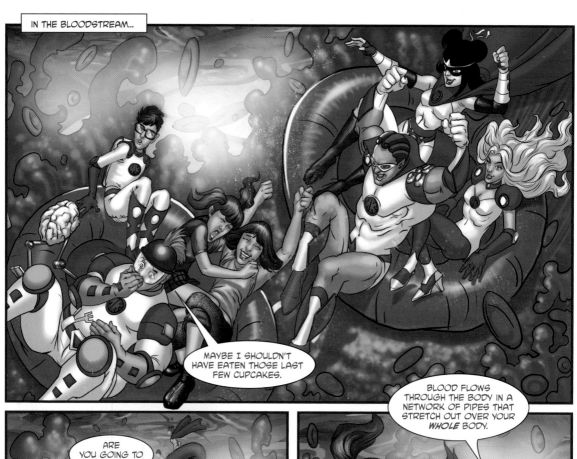

MAYBE I SHOULDN'T HAVE EATEN THOSE LAST FEW CUPCAKES.

BLOOD FLOWS THROUGH THE BODY IN A NETWORK OF PIPES THAT STRETCH OUT OVER YOUR *WHOLE* BODY.

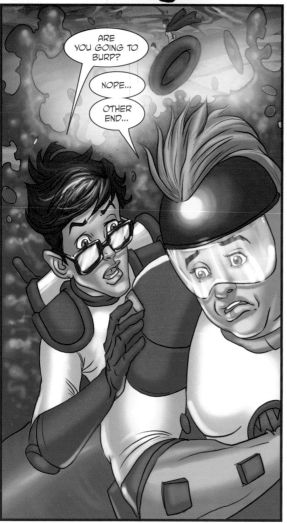

ARE YOU GOING TO BURP?

NOPE...

OTHER END...

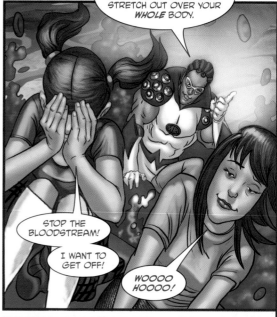

STOP THE BLOODSTREAM! I WANT TO GET OFF!

WOOOO HOOOO!

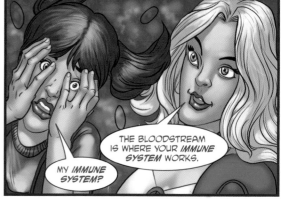

THE BLOODSTREAM IS WHERE YOUR *IMMUNE SYSTEM* WORKS.

MY *IMMUNE SYSTEM?*

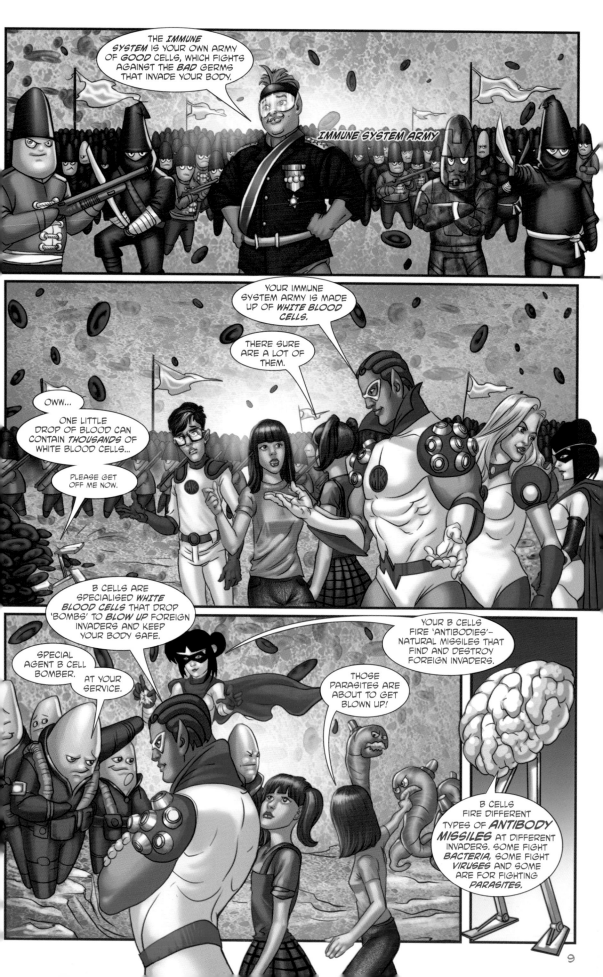

9

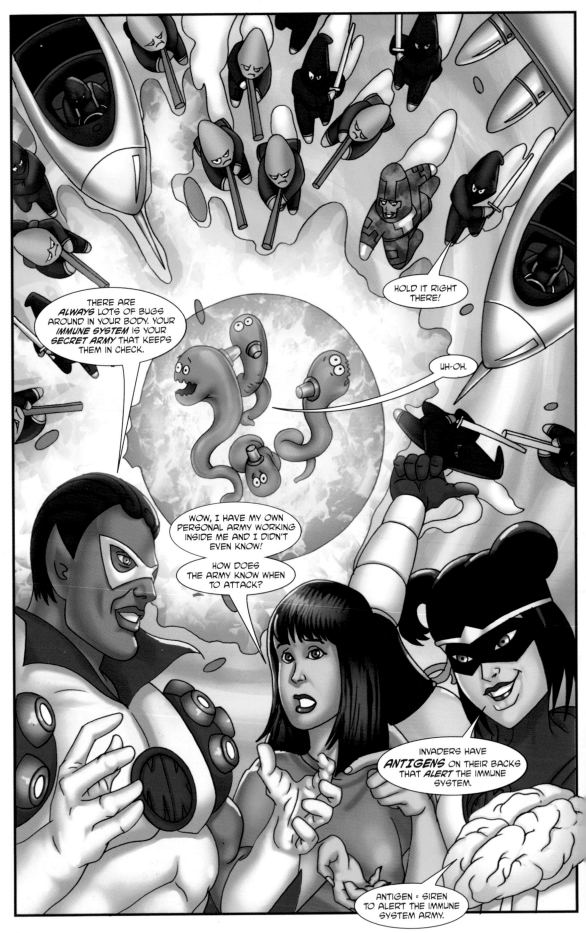

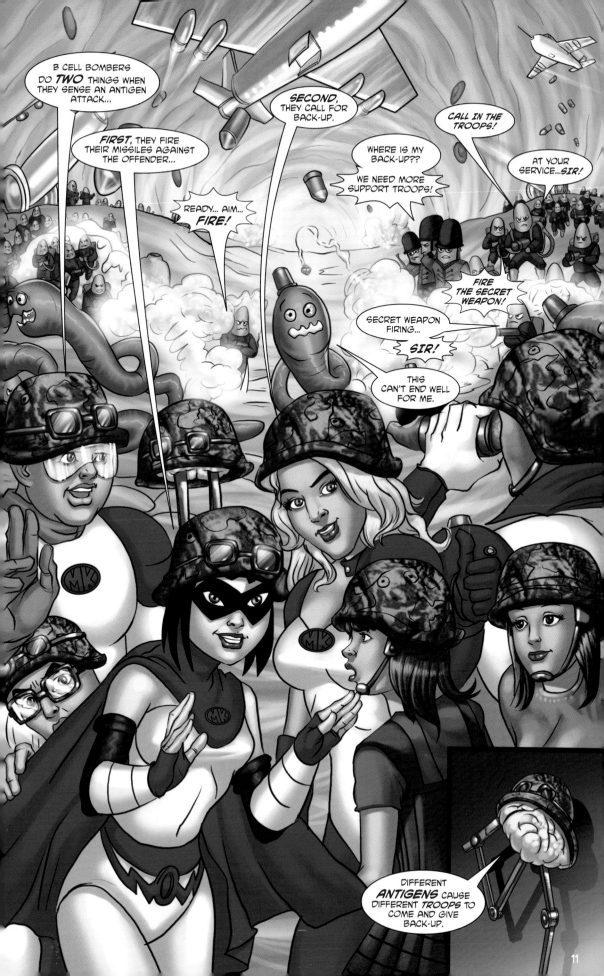

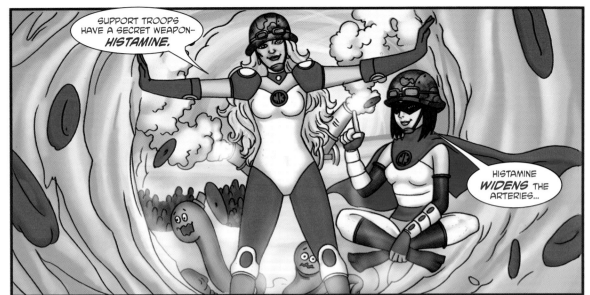

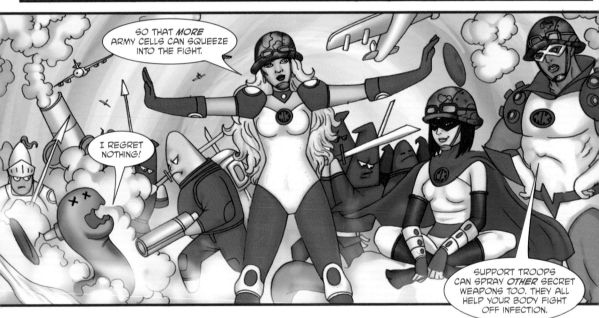

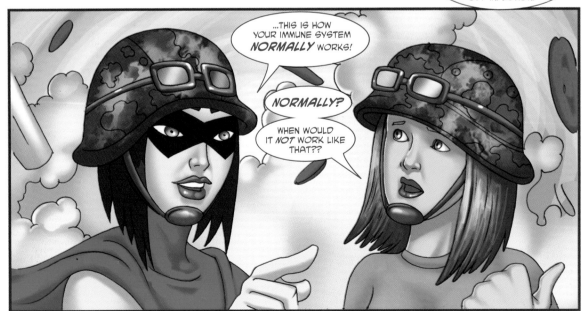

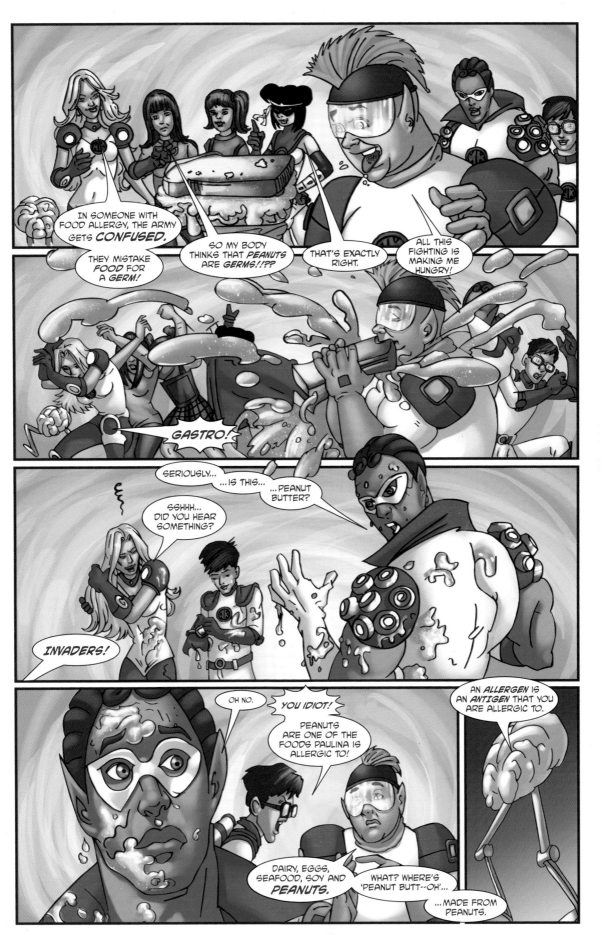

IN SOMEONE WITH FOOD ALLERGY, THE ARMY GETS *CONFUSED.*

THEY MISTAKE *FOOD* FOR A *GERM!*

SO MY BODY THINKS THAT *PEANUTS* ARE *GERMS!!??*

THAT'S EXACTLY RIGHT.

ALL THIS FIGHTING IS MAKING ME HUNGRY!

GASTRO!

SERIOUSLY...

...IS THIS...

...PEANUT BUTTER?

SSHHH... DID YOU HEAR SOMETHING?

INVADERS!

OH NO.

YOU IDIOT!

PEANUTS ARE ONE OF THE FOODS PAULINA IS ALLERGIC TO!

AN *ALLERGEN* IS AN *ANTIGEN* THAT YOU ARE ALLERGIC TO.

DAIRY, EGGS, SEAFOOD, SOY AND *PEANUTS.*

WHAT? WHERE'S 'PEANUT BUTT--OH'...

...MADE FROM PEANUTS.

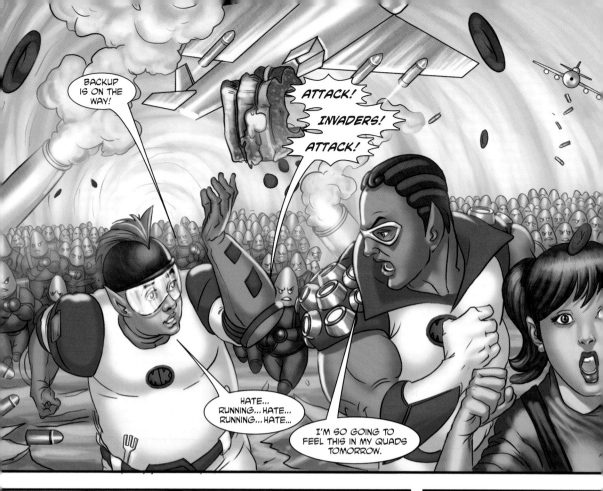

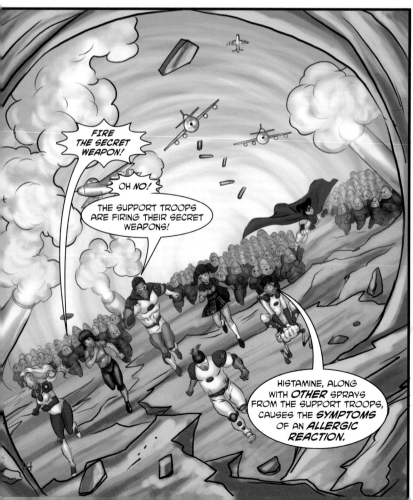

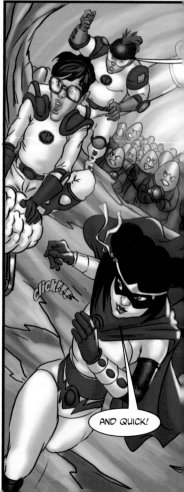

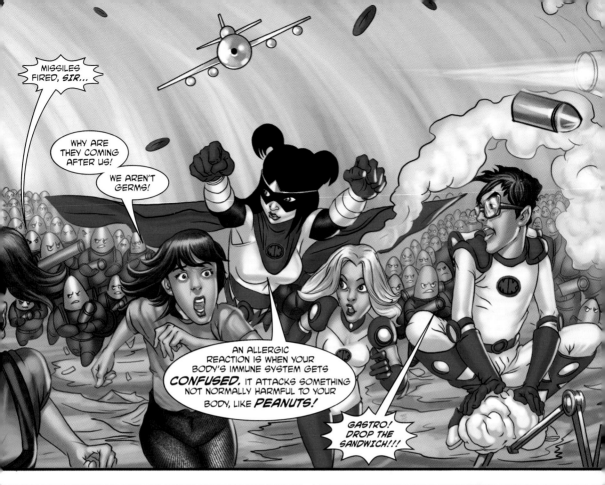
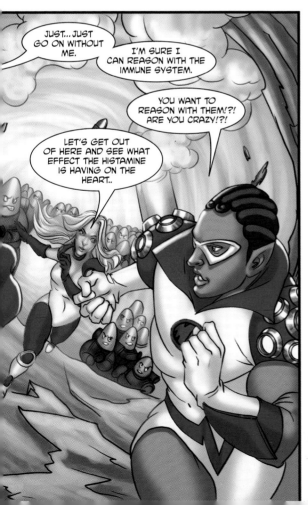
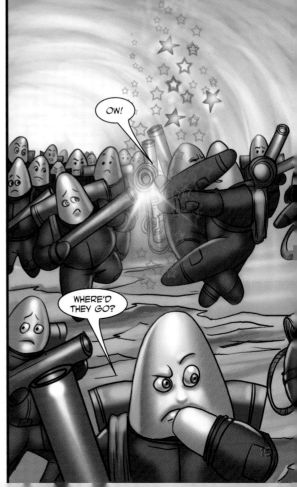

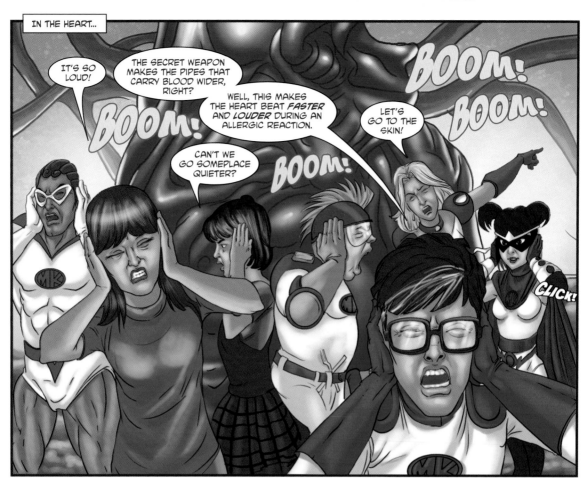

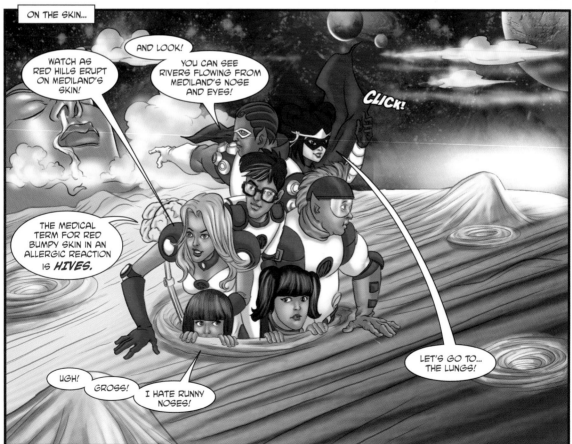

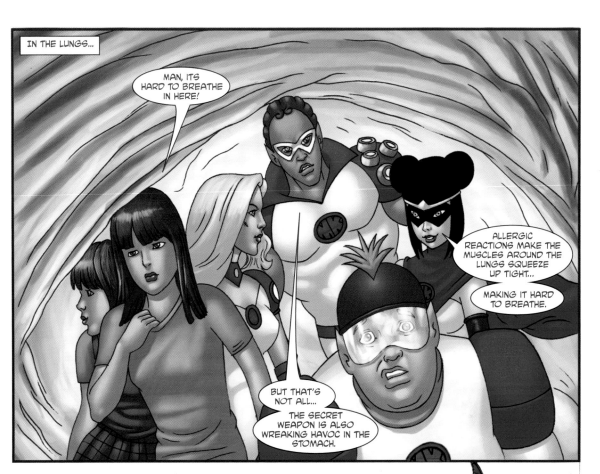

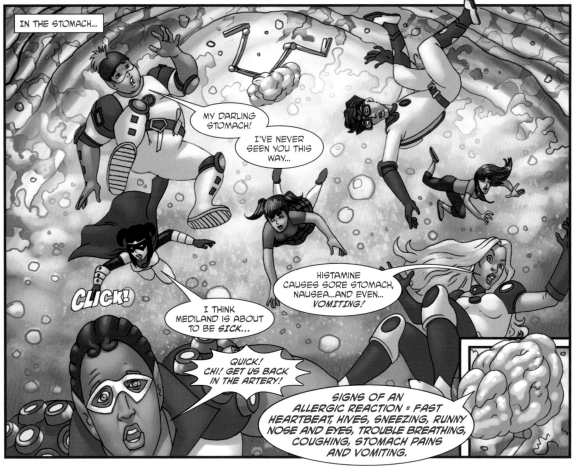

CLICK!

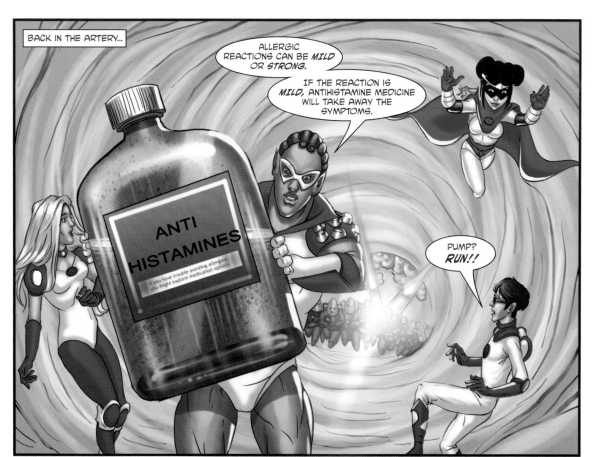

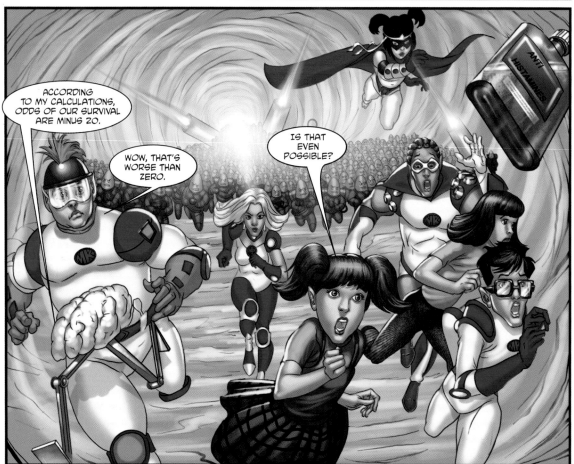

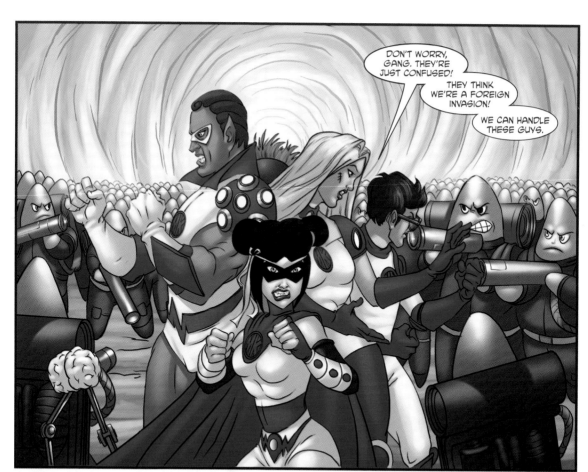

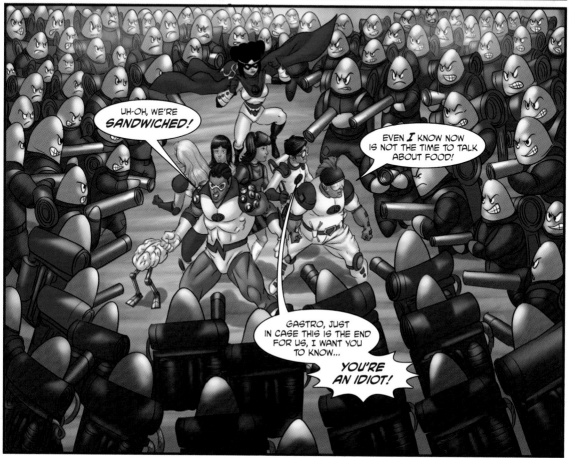

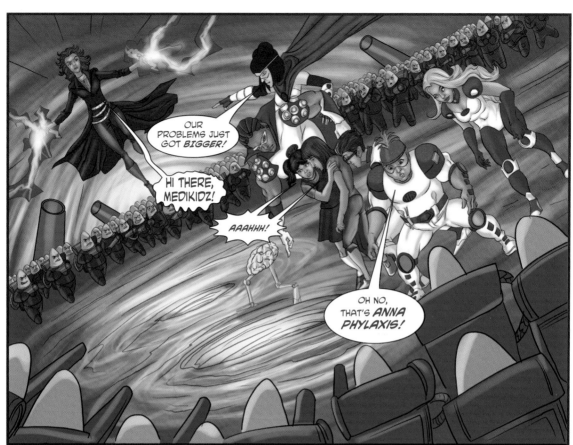

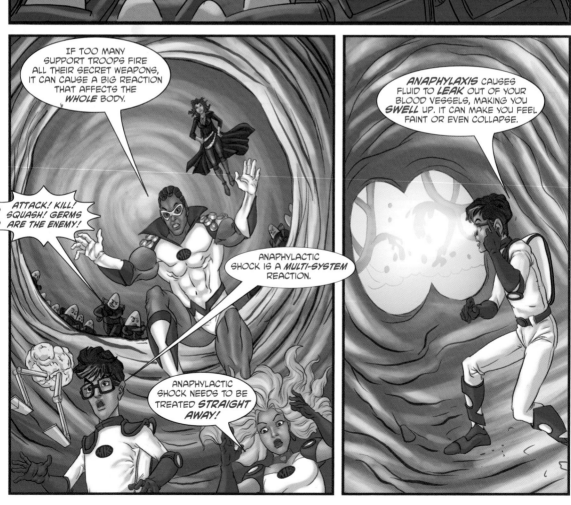

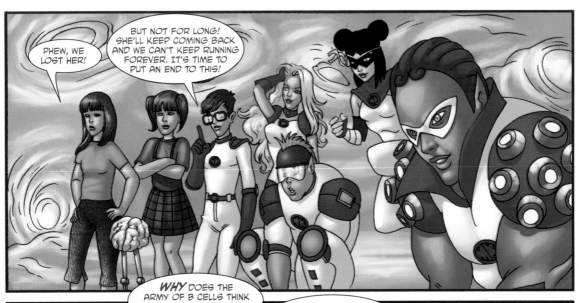

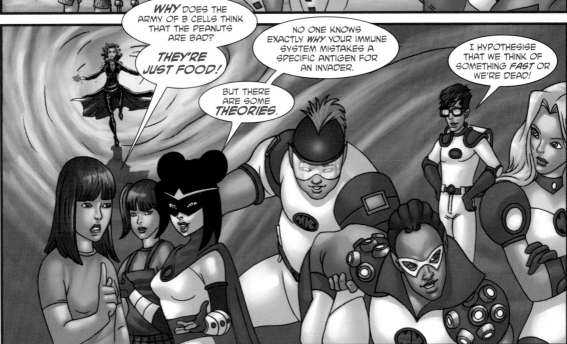

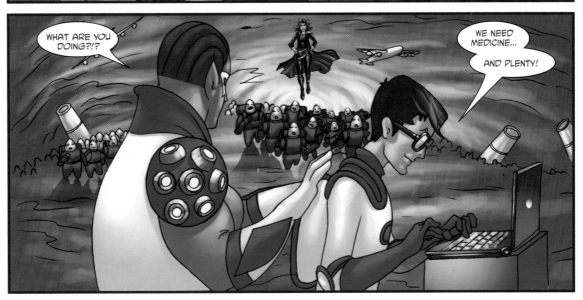

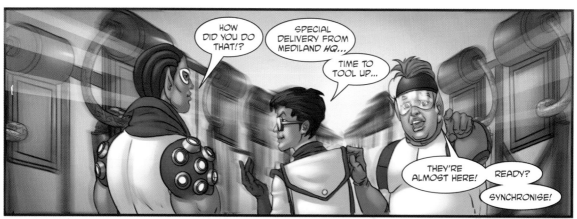

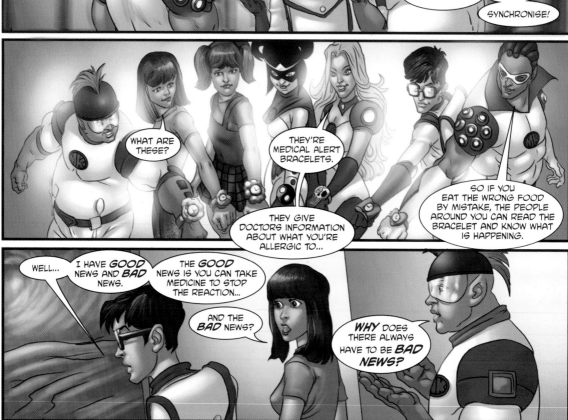

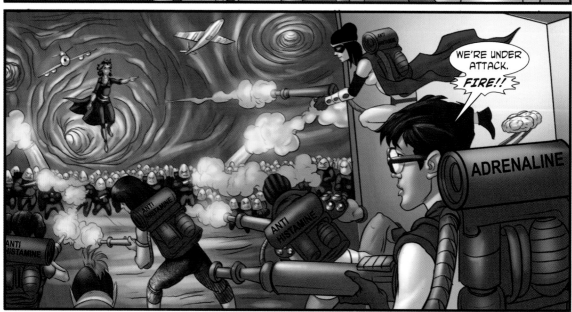

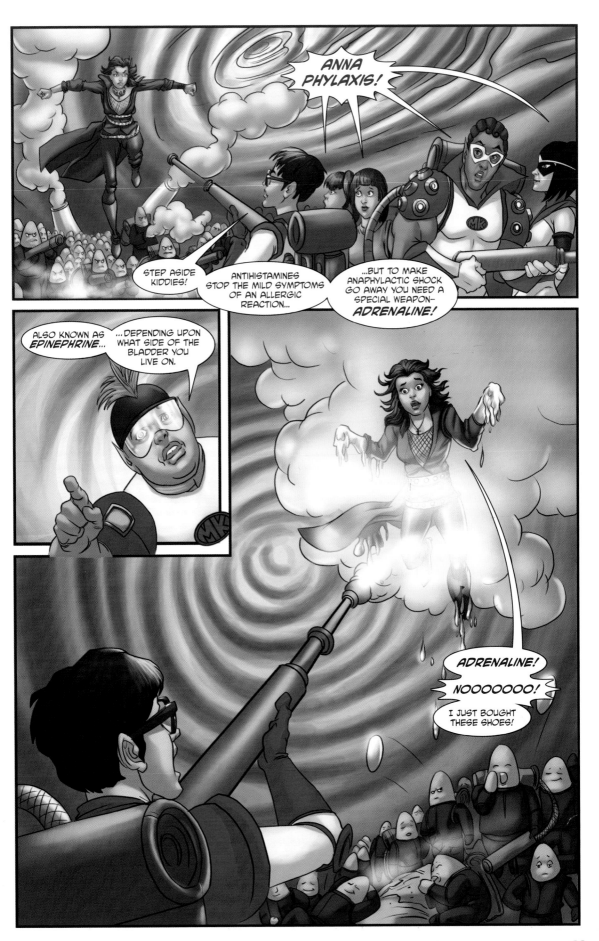

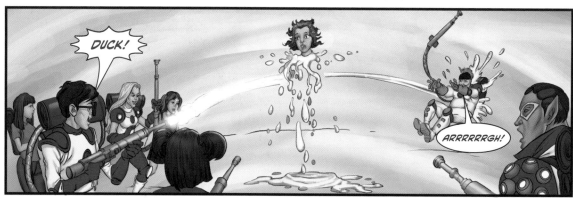

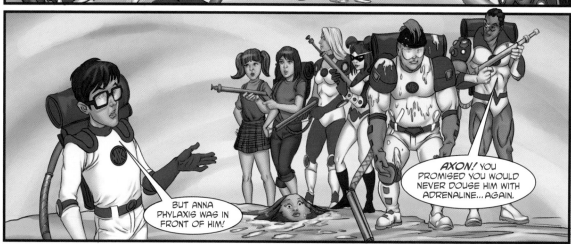

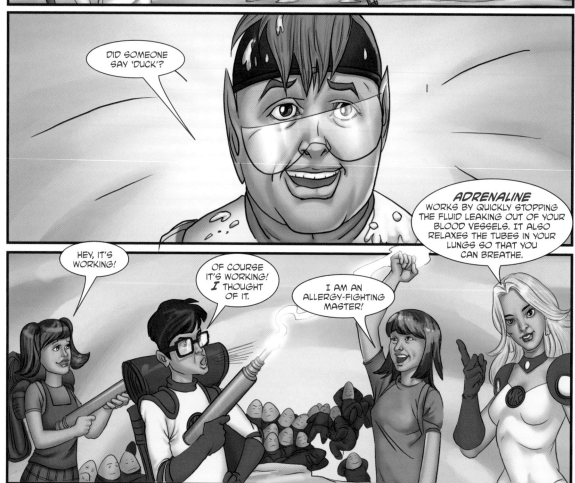

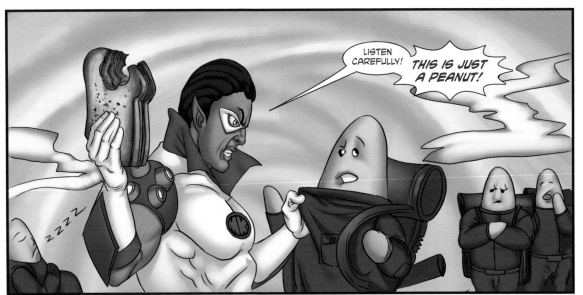

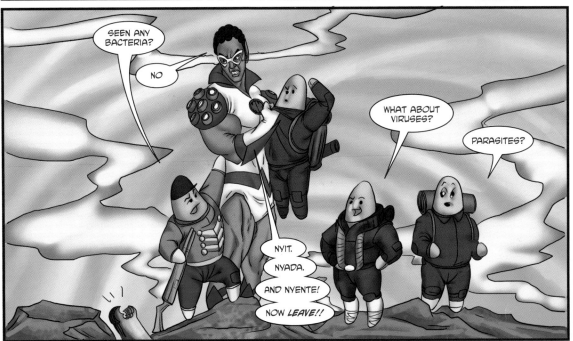

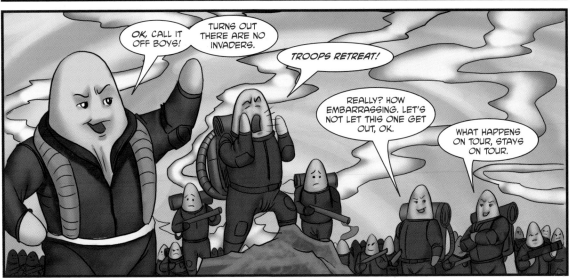

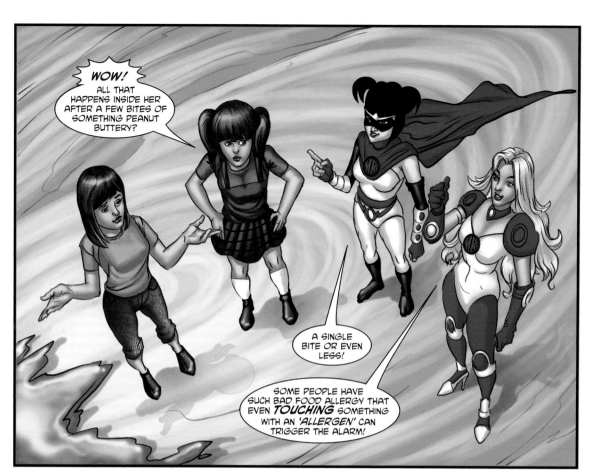

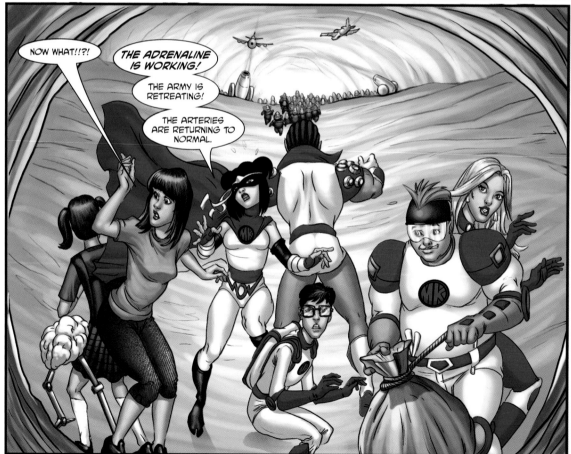

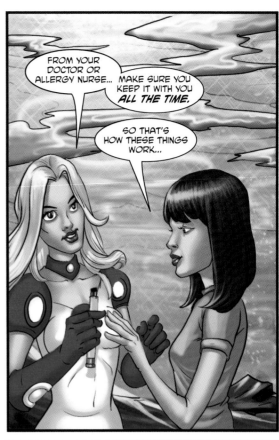

ADRENALINE IS AWESOME!

HOW DO I GET SOME OF THAT?!?

FROM YOUR DOCTOR OR ALLERGY NURSE... MAKE SURE YOU KEEP IT WITH YOU *ALL THE TIME.*

SO THAT'S HOW THESE THINGS WORK...

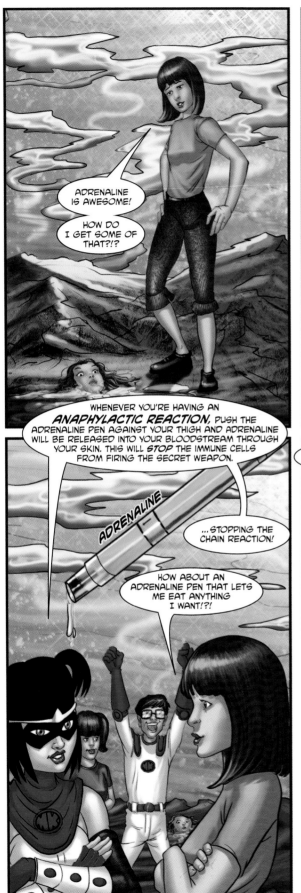

WHENEVER YOU'RE HAVING AN *ANAPHYLACTIC REACTION,* PUSH THE ADRENALINE PEN AGAINST YOUR THIGH AND ADRENALINE WILL BE RELEASED INTO YOUR BLOODSTREAM THROUGH YOUR SKIN. THIS WILL *STOP* THE IMMUNE CELLS FROM FIRING THE SECRET WEAPON.

ADRENALINE

...STOPPING THE CHAIN REACTION!

HOW ABOUT AN ADRENALINE PEN THAT LETS ME EAT ANYTHING I WANT!?!

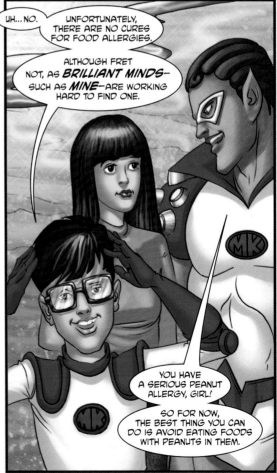

UH... NO.

UNFORTUNATELY, THERE ARE NO CURES FOR FOOD ALLERGIES.

ALTHOUGH FRET NOT, AS *BRILLIANT MINDS*— SUCH AS *MINE*—ARE WORKING HARD TO FIND ONE.

YOU HAVE A SERIOUS PEANUT ALLERGY, GIRL!

SO FOR NOW, THE BEST THING YOU CAN DO IS AVOID EATING FOODS WITH PEANUTS IN THEM.

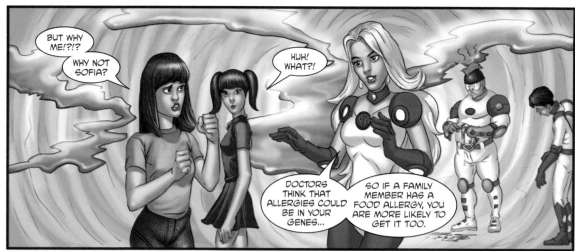

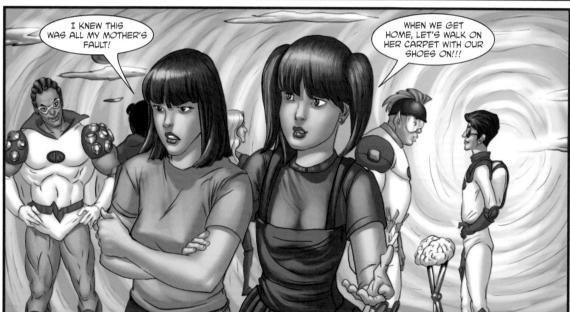

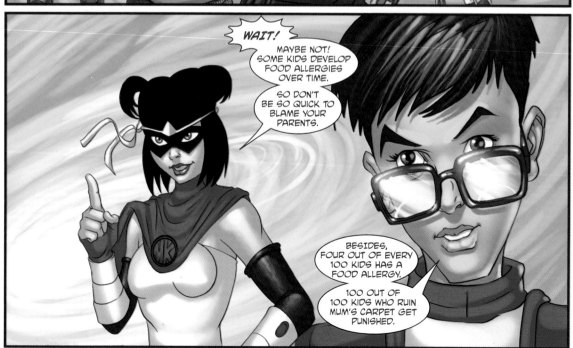

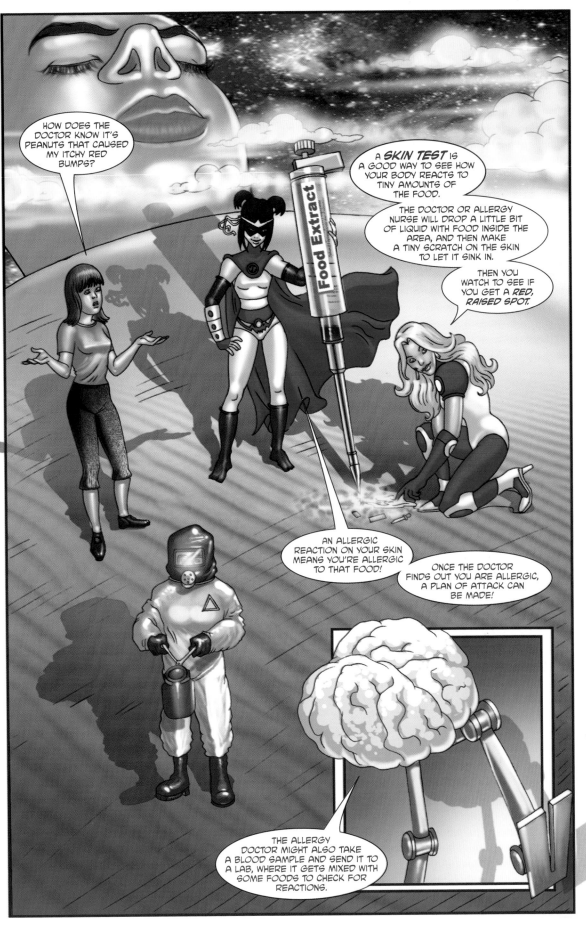

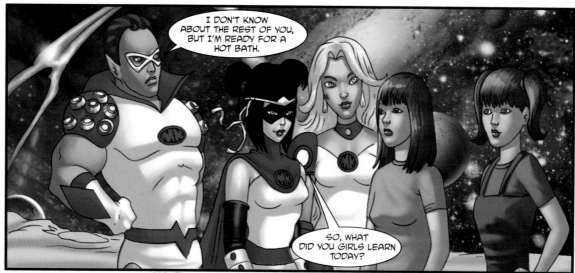

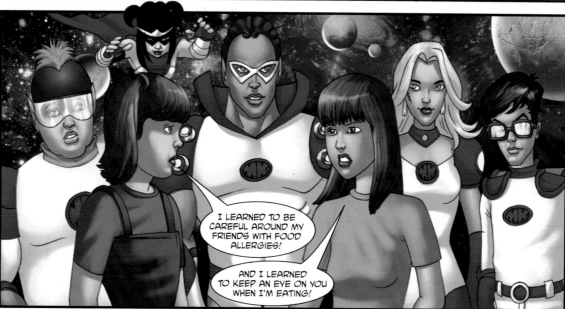

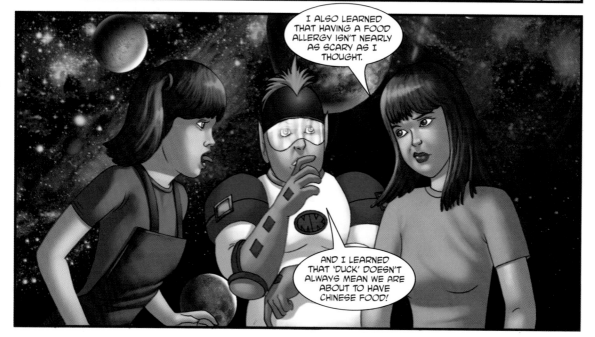

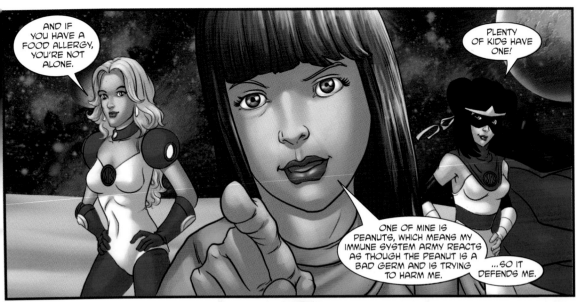

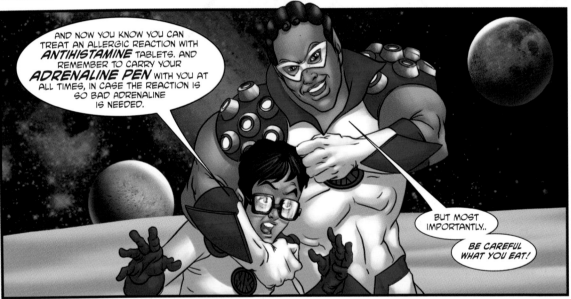

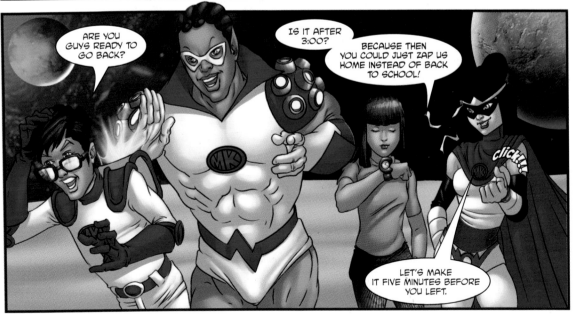

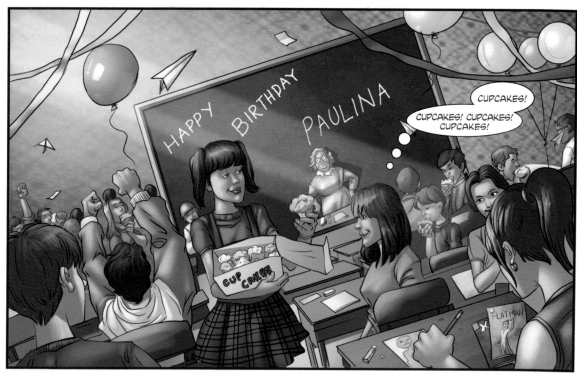

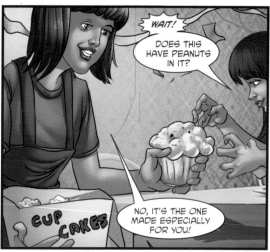

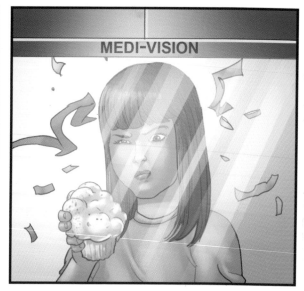

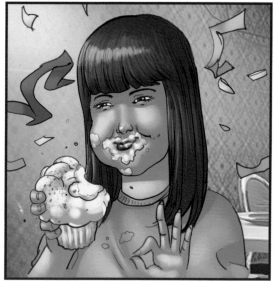

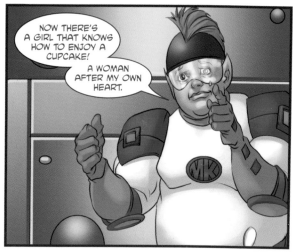